I0100425

You Are Nature

Ayurveda for Babies

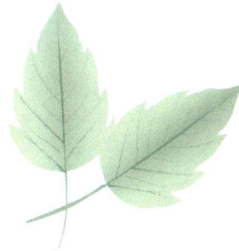

Written and Illustrated by:
Catalina Arango

Copyright © 2025 Catalina Arango
All rights reserved.
No part of this book may be reproduced or transmitted in any
form without written permission from the publisher.
Published by Awaken Prana Press
Miami, Florida
ISBN (paperback): 979-8-9941052-1-4
ISBN (hardcover): 979-8-9941052-0-7
Illustrations by Catalina Arango

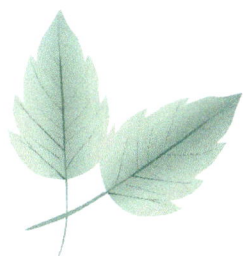

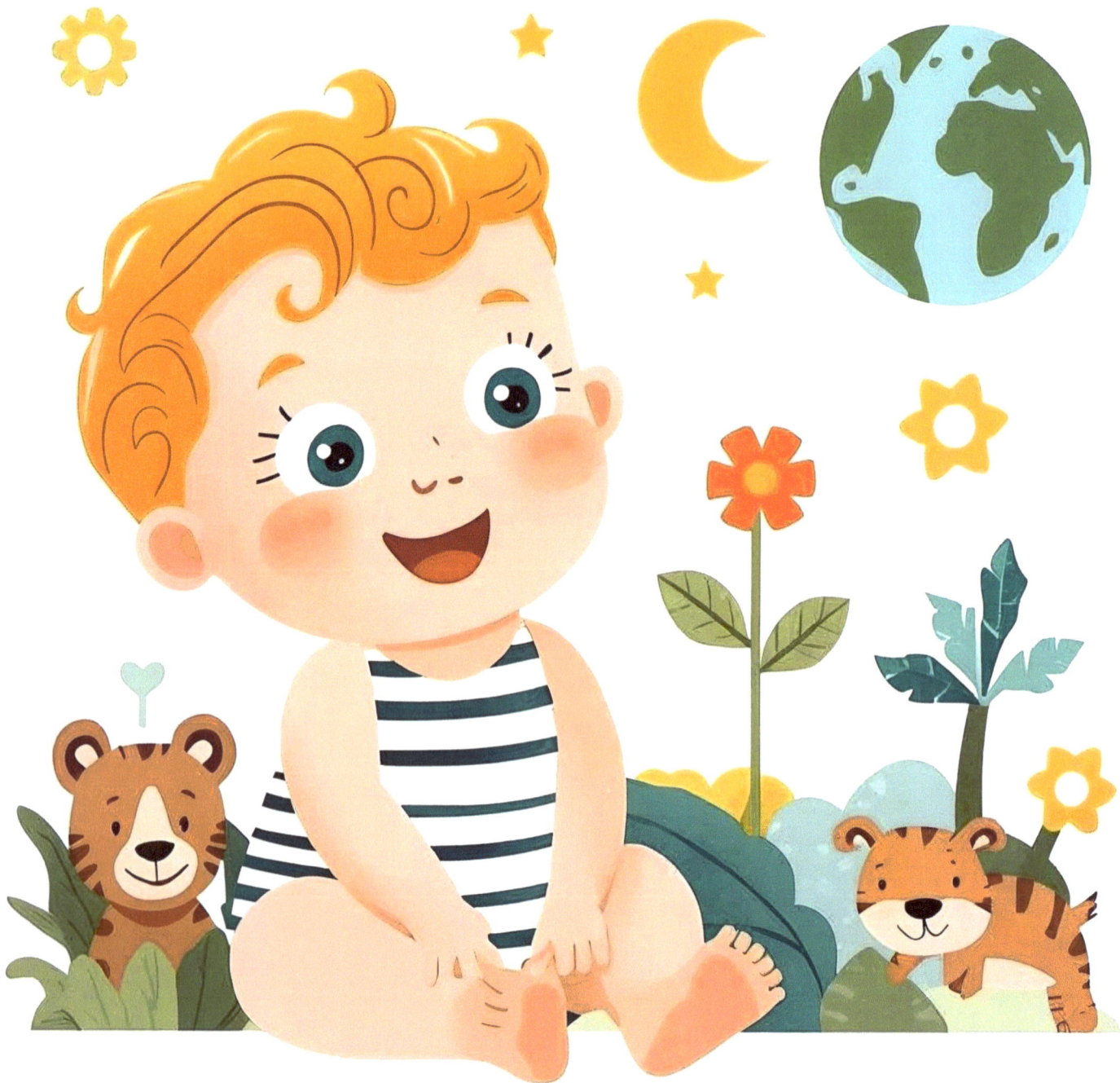

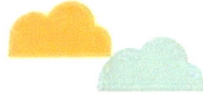

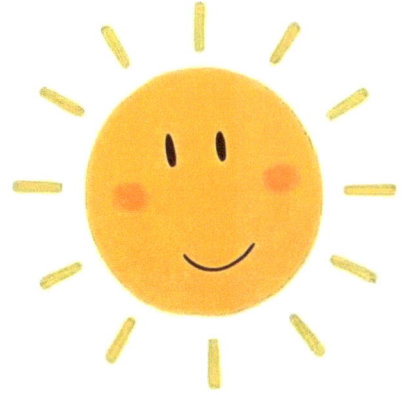

Hi, baby!
You are a tiny part
of this BIG
beautiful world.

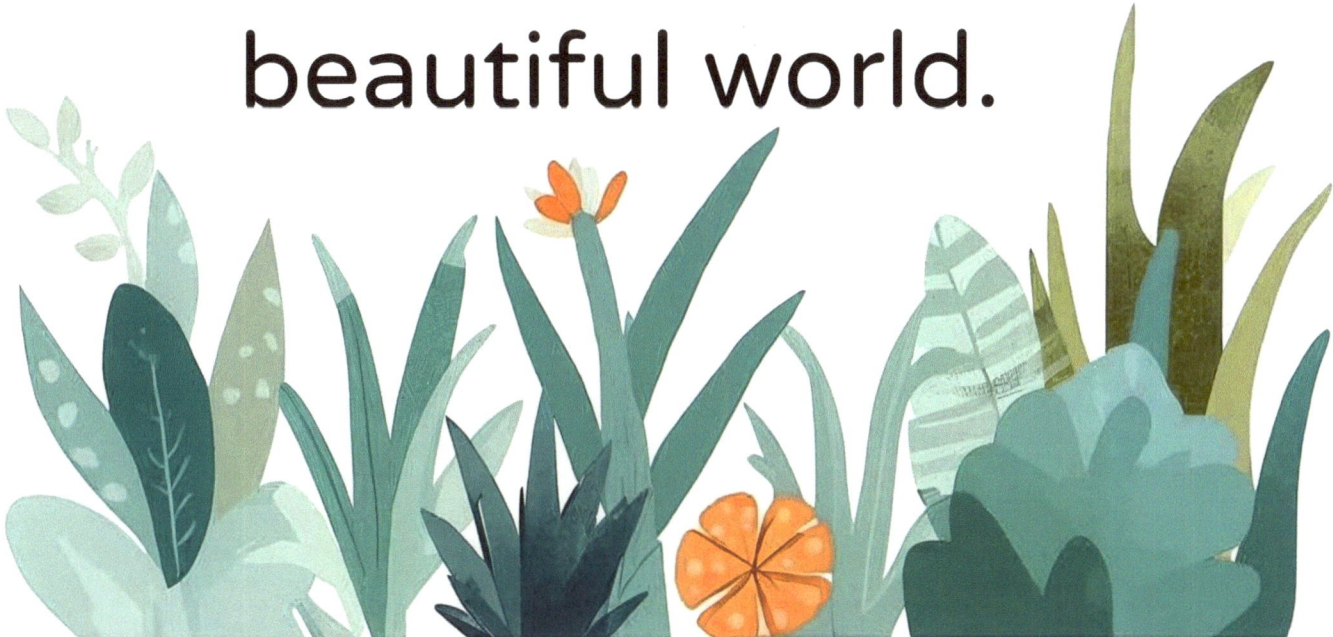

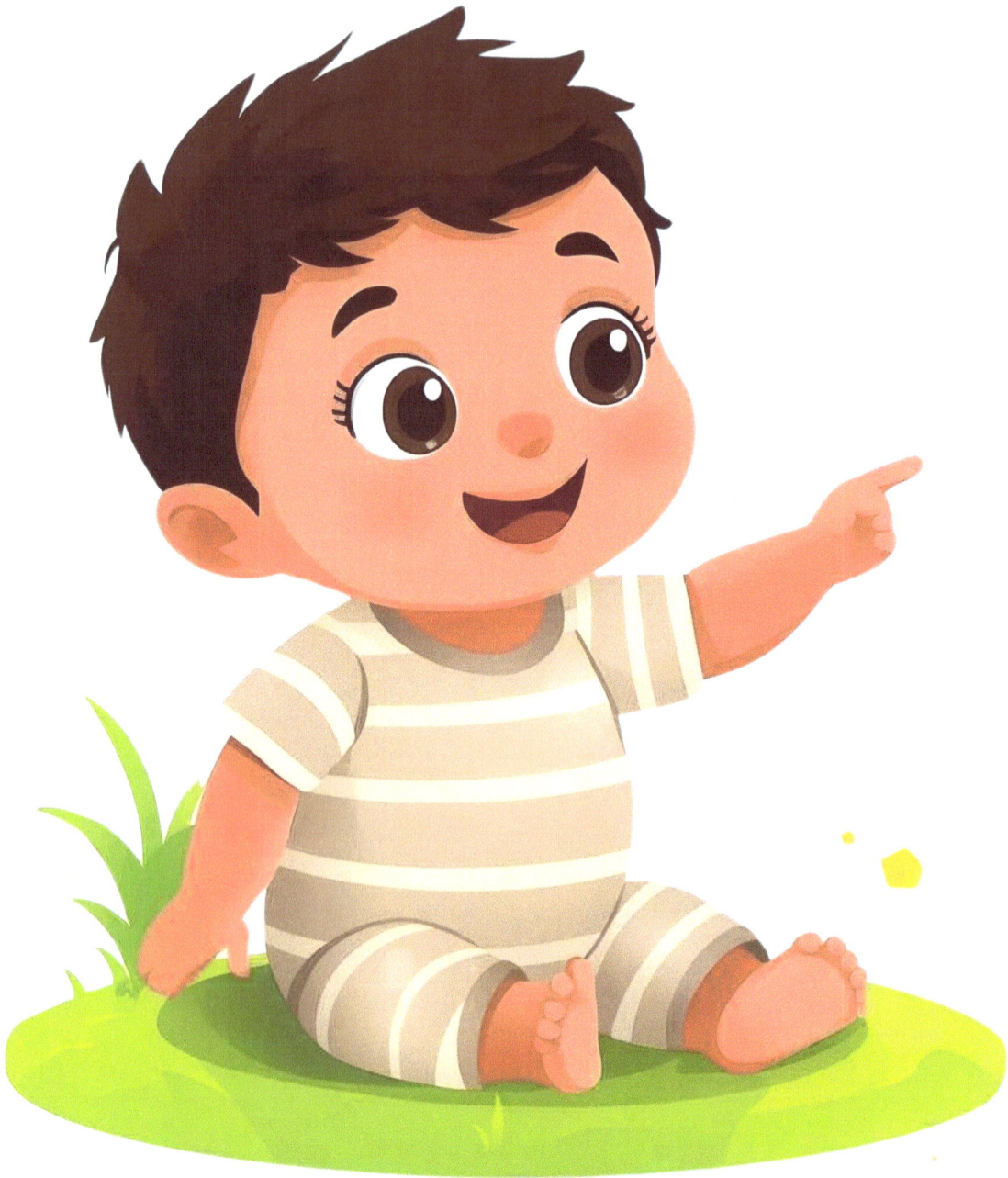

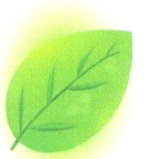

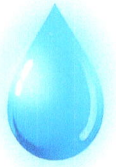

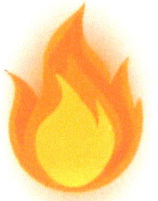

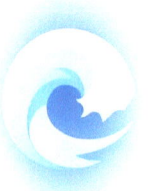

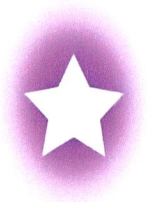

You are made of

🍃 Earth, 💧 Water,
🔥 Fire, 🌀 Air and
⭐ Space –

Just like
everything else!

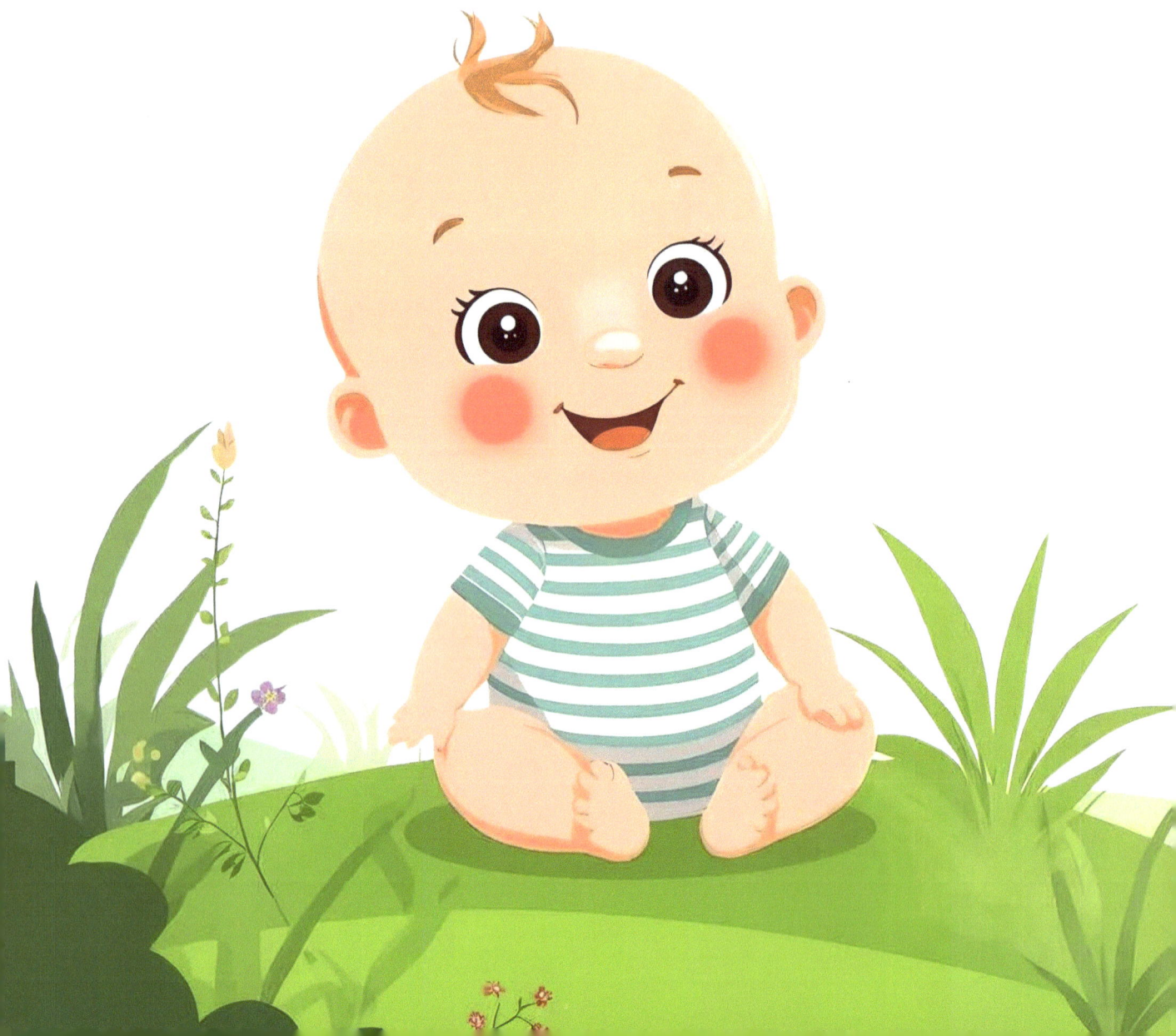

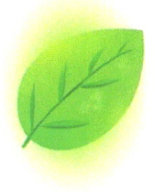

Squishy belly, chunky legs—

That's Earth!

Strong. Steady. Safe.

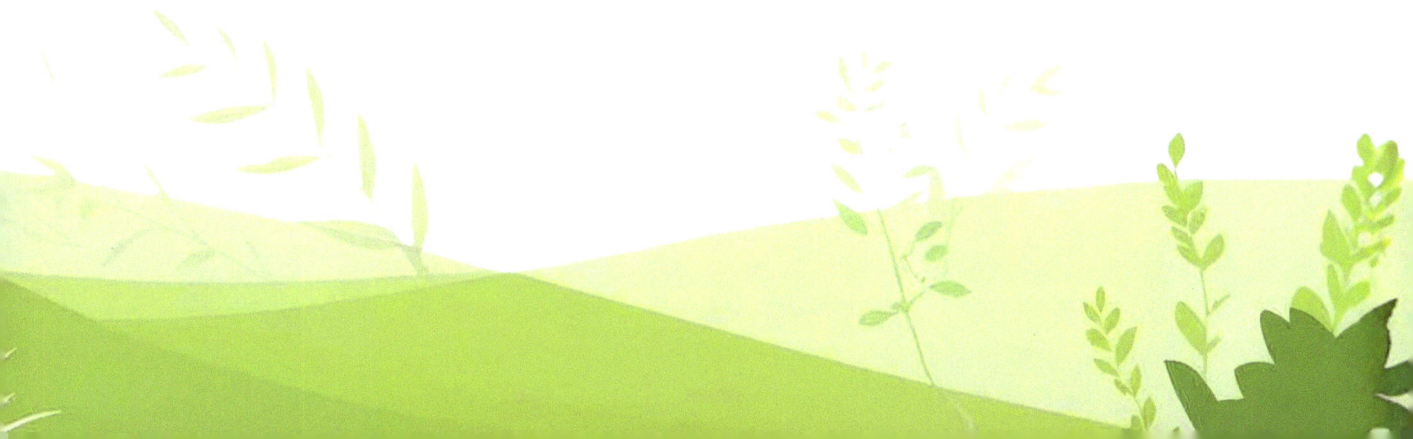

Drool and milk and tears—

That's Water!

Cool. Soft. Smooth.

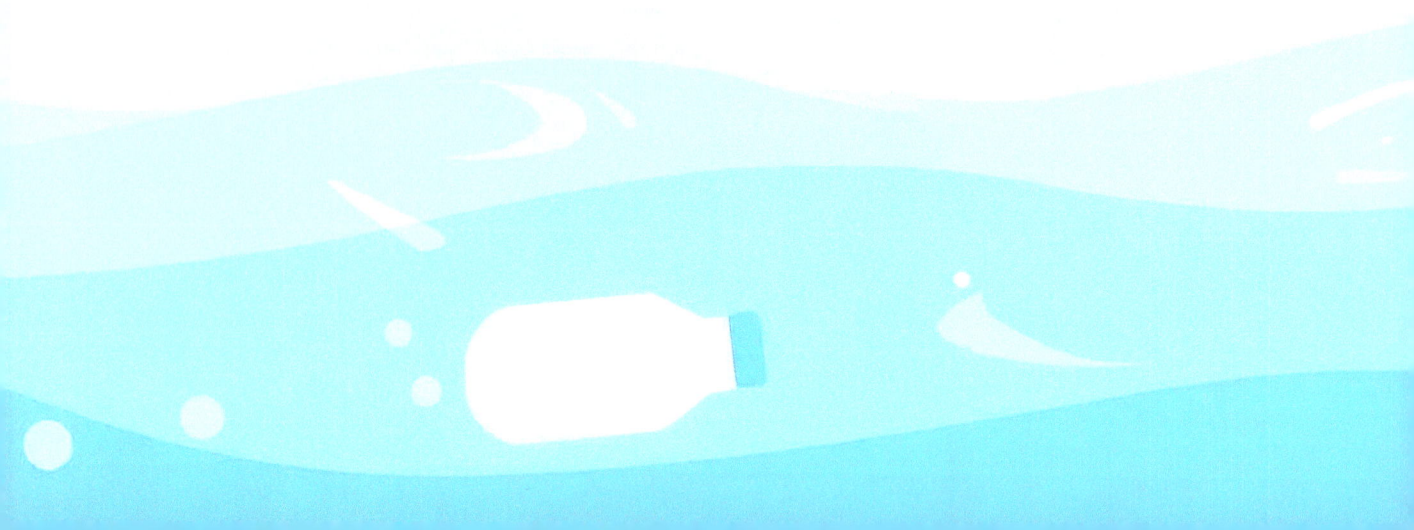

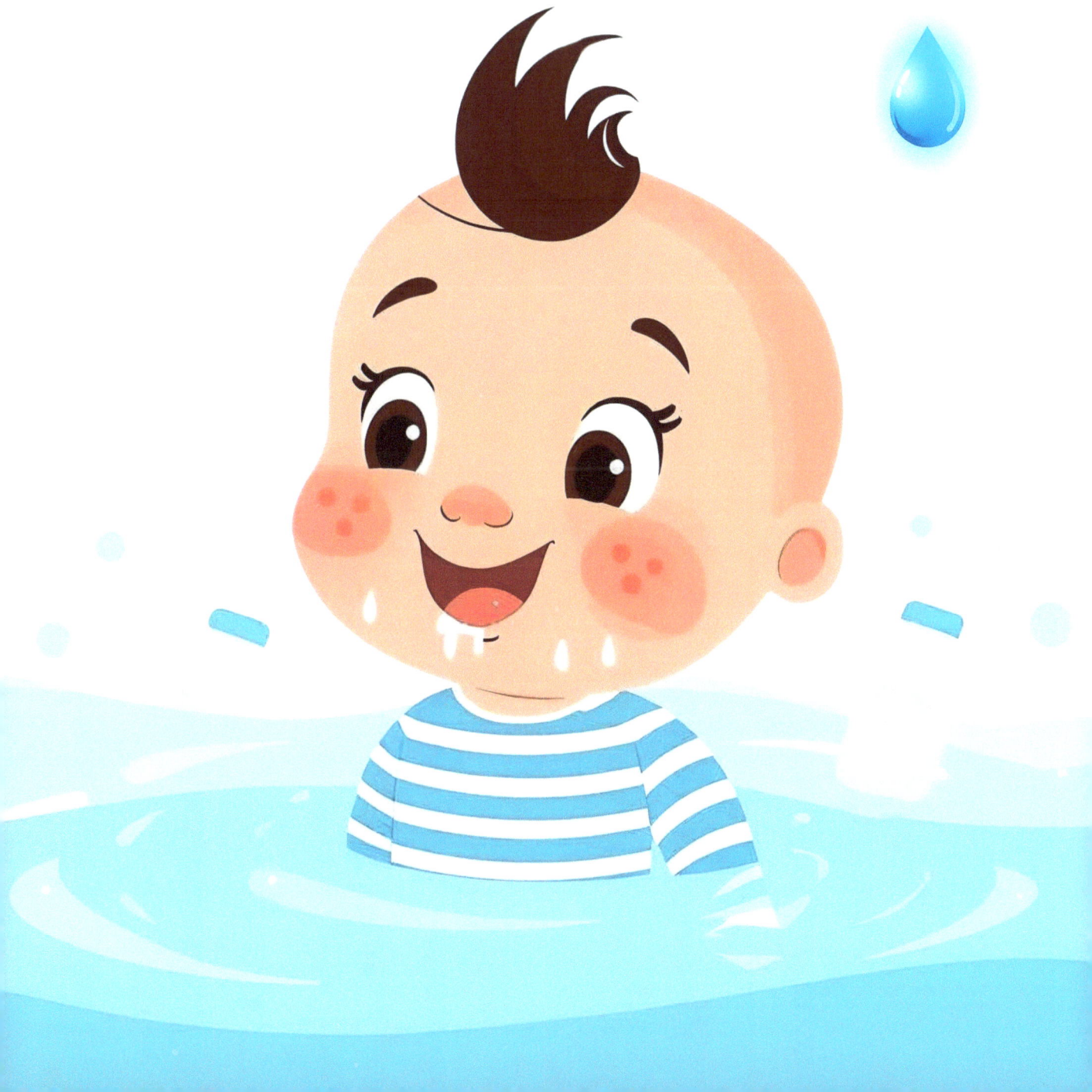

Warm belly, bright eyes—

That's Fire!

Warm. Happy. Hungry.

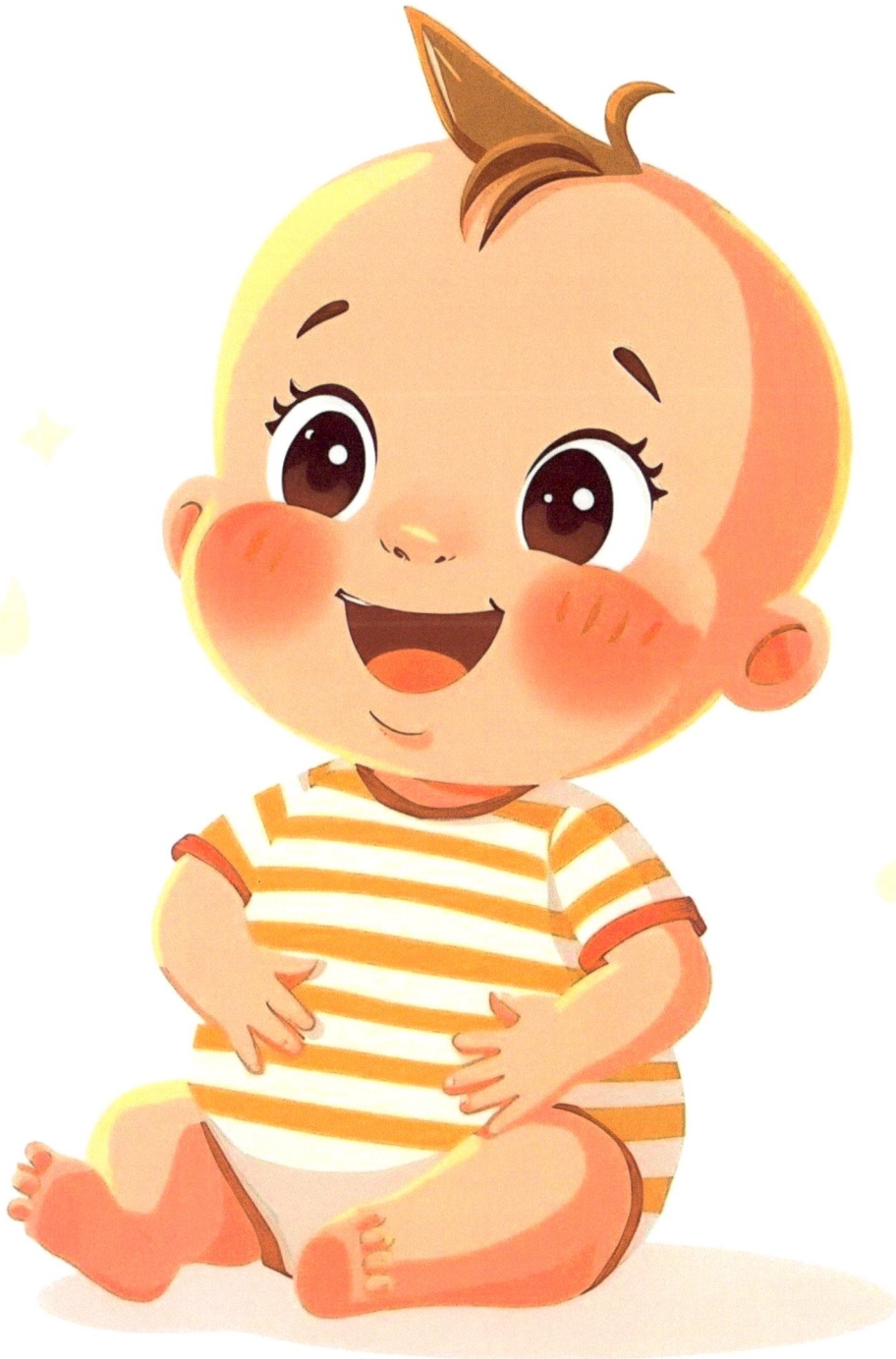

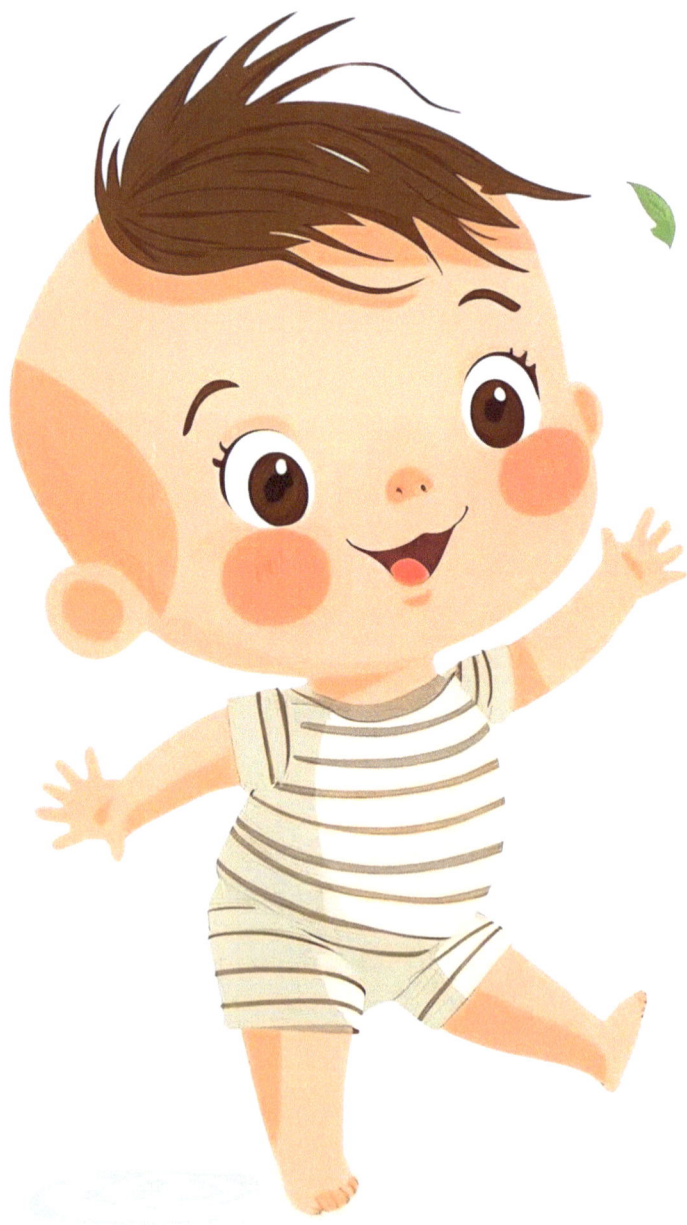

Kick, wiggle, spin—

That's Air!

Fast. Light. Fun.

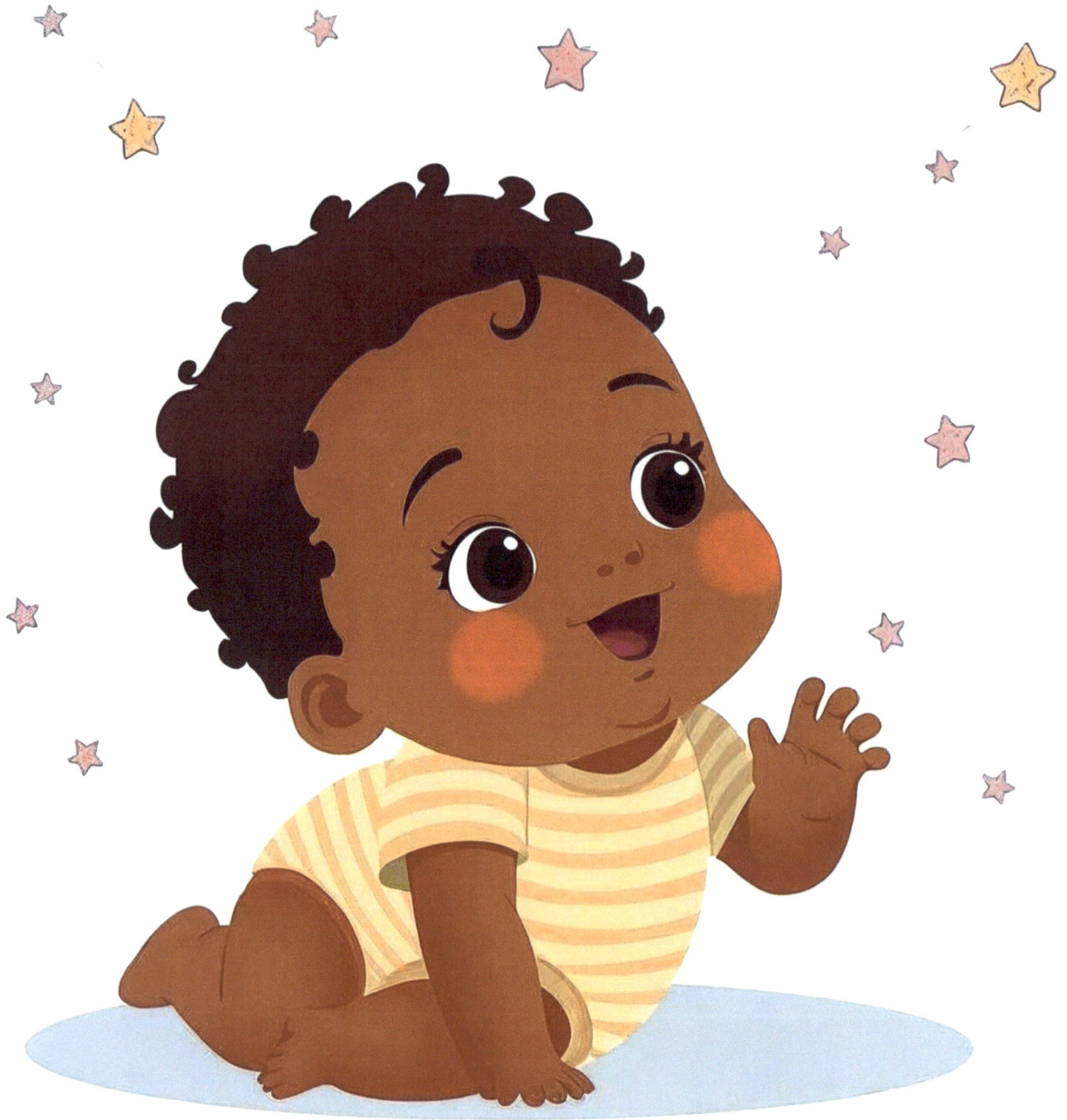

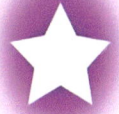

Quiet moments, a breath—

That's Space.

Still. Open. Wide.

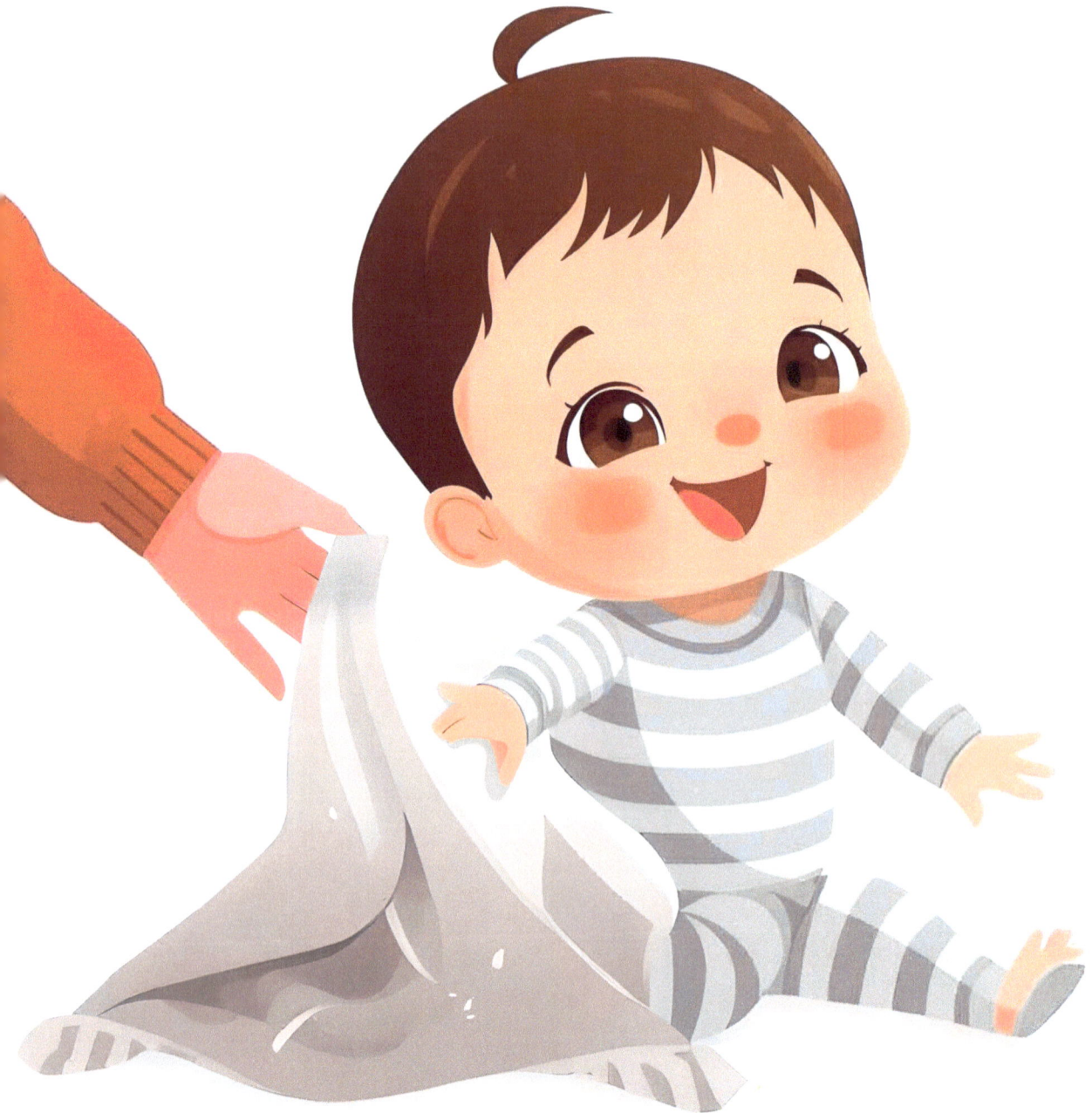

Cool loves cool.
Wiggle loves wiggle.

But sometimes...
Too much "same" feels icky.

So we add the opposite to
bring balance.

Mornings are for waking.
Afternoons are for playing.
Evenings are for cuddles.
Nights are for rest.

Your body loves rhythm.

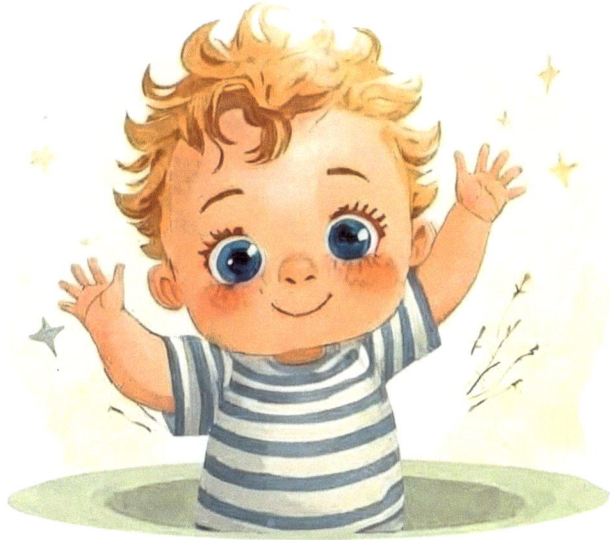

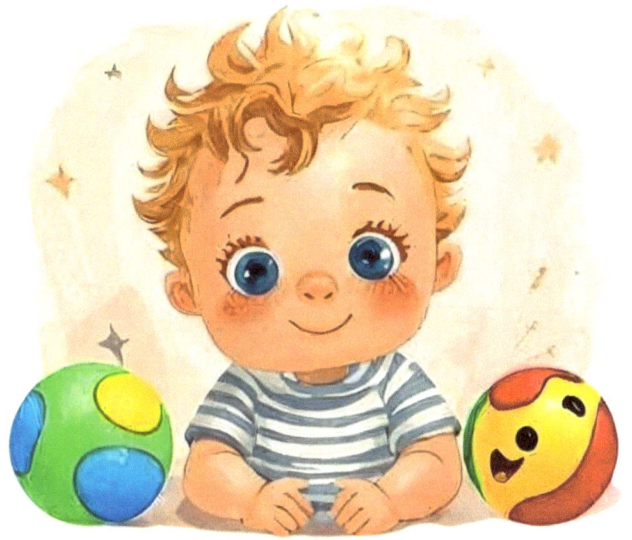

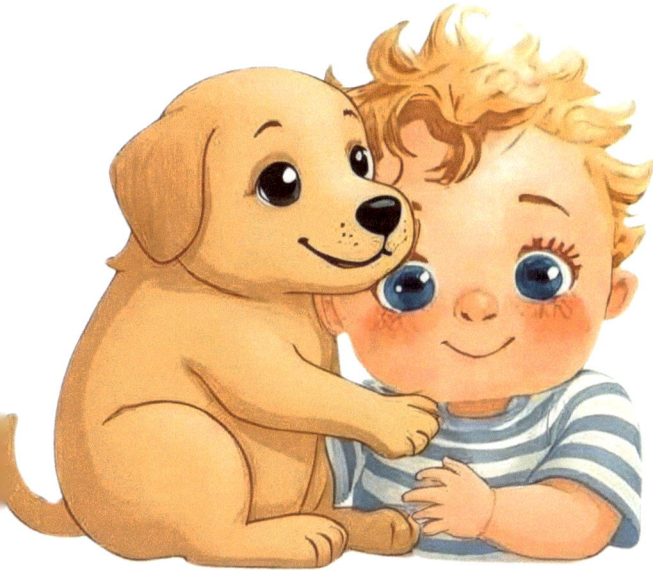

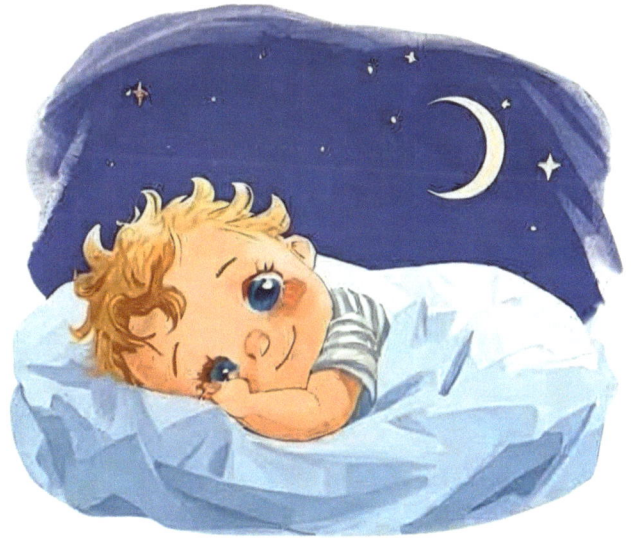

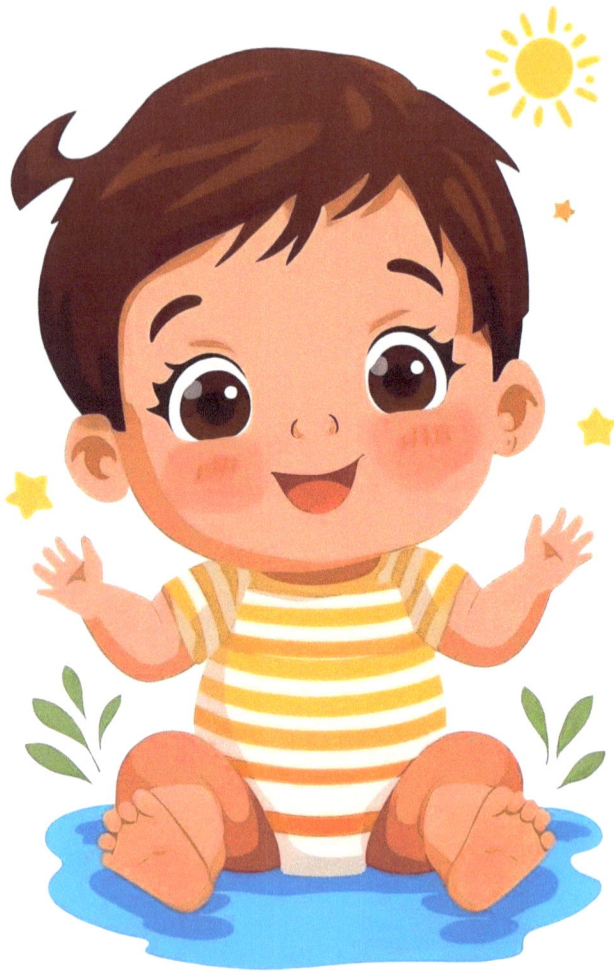

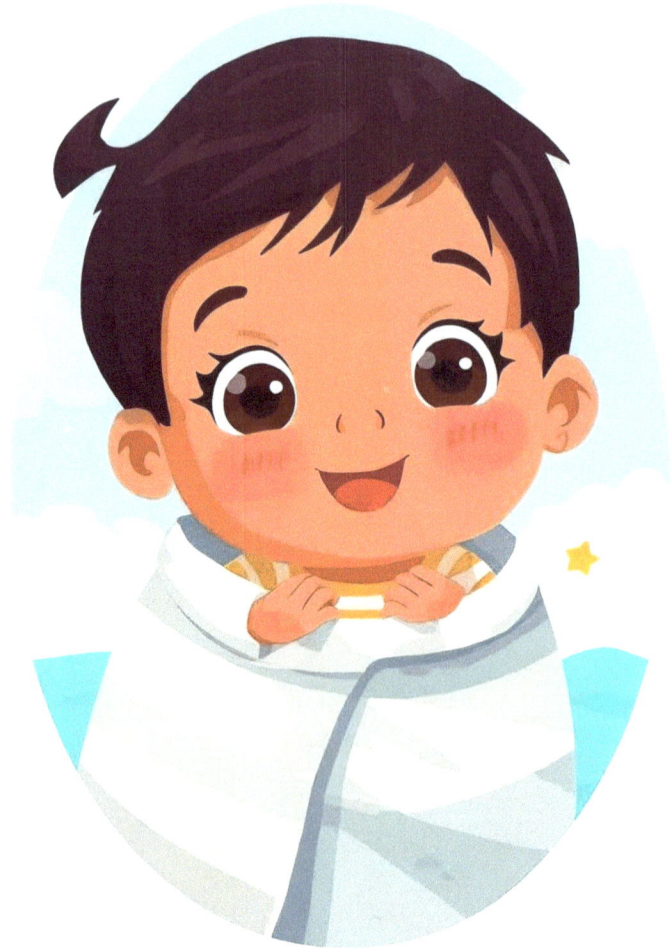

When it's hot, we cool you.

When it's cold, we warm you.

When the world shifts, we shift with it.

You are made of
nature.

You already know
what to do.

We're just here
to help you grow.

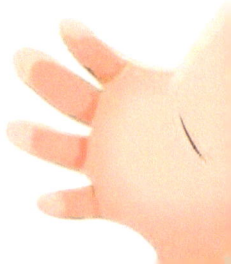

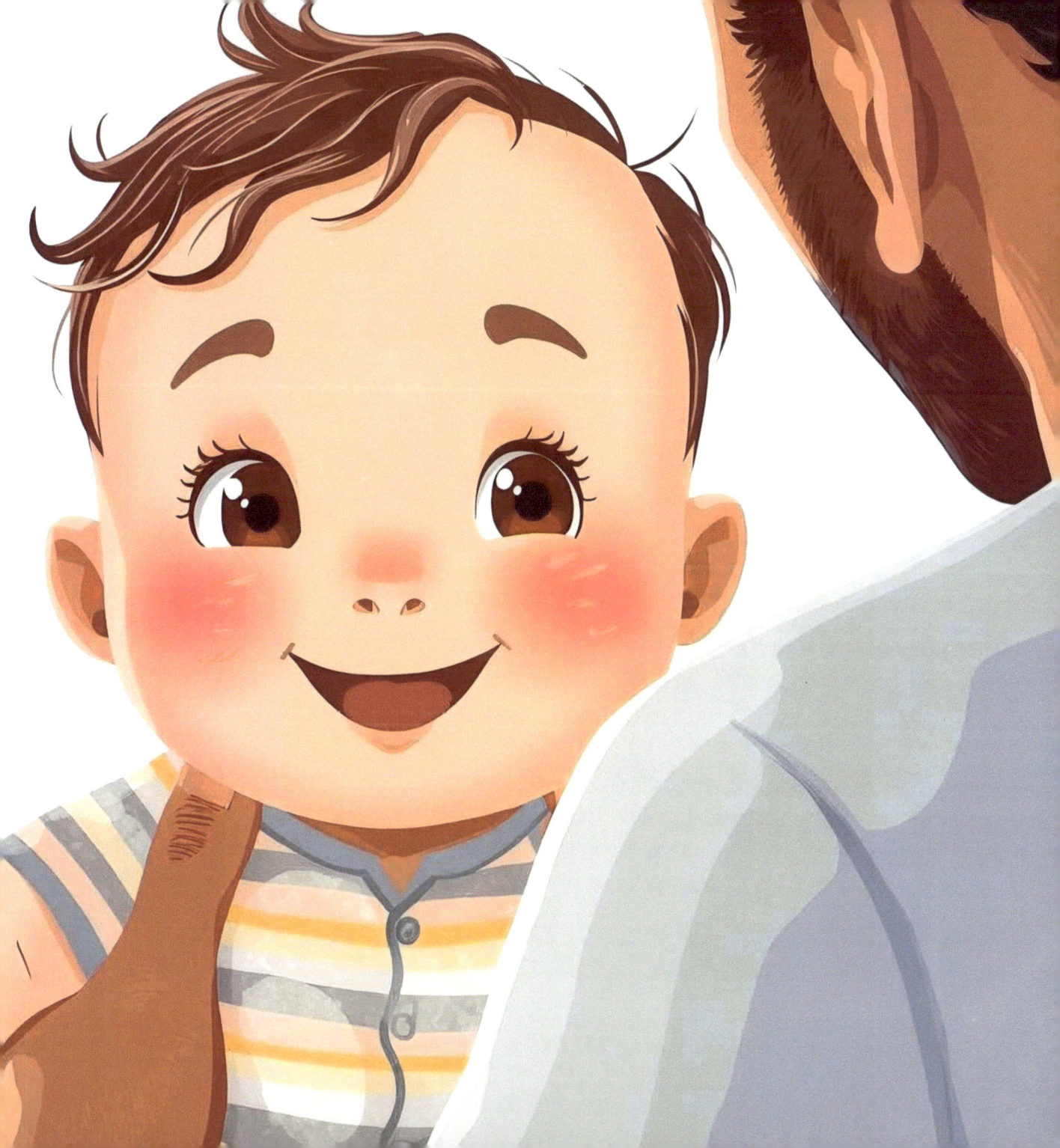

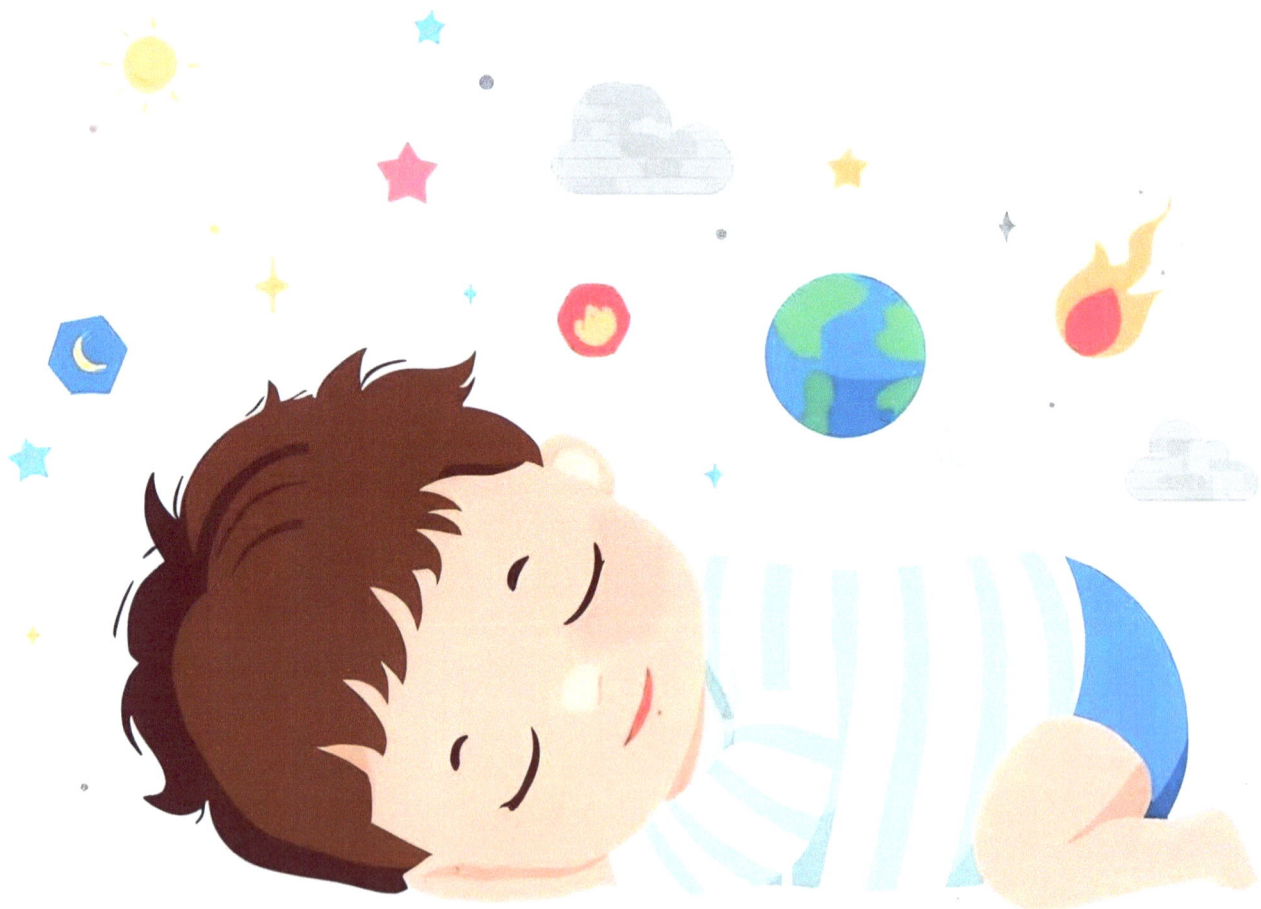

Earth holds you.
Water rocks you.
Fire keeps you warm.
Air whispers songs.
And space lets you dream.

Goodnight, baby.
Goodnight.

Parent's Note

Ayurveda teaches that every child is part of nature—made of the elements and guided by simple rhythms. This book uses gentle words and images to help your baby notice sensations, routines, and the world around them.

As you read, point to the pictures, repeat the sounds, and enjoy the moment. Let this be a small reminder to slow down, tune in, and honor your baby's natural rhythm.

With love,
Catalina

www.ingramcontent.com/pod-product-compliance
Lightning Source LLC
Chambersburg PA
CBHW040811300326
41914CB00065B/1492